COOKBOOK
FOR
HYPERTENSIVE
PATIENT

Delicious and Healthy
Recipes for a Heart-Healthy Diet

Zakka Shalom

Copyright © 2023 by Zakka Shalom

TABLE OF CONTENTS

INTRODUCTION

Once upon a time, there was a man called Henry who had been living with hypertension for many years. He was very afraid of the potential health risks, and was determined to do something about it. One day, a friend suggested that he try a special diet that was known to help with hypertension. Henry was hesitant at first, but eventually decided to give it a try.

The diet consisted of a lot of fruits and vegetables, as well as lean proteins and whole grains. He was also instructed to cut out all fried foods, processed sugars, and any type of processed food. At first, Henry was sceptical. He thought he would never be able to stick to such a strict diet. But over time, he found that he was actually enjoying the food he was eating and was finding it easy to stick with the plan.

With the help of this diet, Henry's hypertension began to slowly improve. He was able to make lifestyle changes to help reduce stress, such as getting more exercise and relaxation techniques.

After a few months, Henry's blood pressure had returned to normal and he was no longer living in fear of the potential health risks of hypertension. He was so thankful to have found a way to overcome his condition.

CHAPTER ONE

Understanding Hypertension

Hypertension, also known as high blood pressure, is a serious condition that affects millions of people around the world. It occurs when the force of blood flowing through the arteries is too high, placing strain on the cardiovascular system and potentially leading to organ damage. Many of the risk factors for hypertension are lifestyle-related, such as being overweight, eating an unhealthy diet, smoking, and not getting enough physical activity. However, there are also certain medical conditions, such as kidney disease and diabetes that can increase a person's risk of developing hypertension.

It is important to learn about the causes, symptoms, and treatments of hypertension, as well as how to prevent it, in order to reduce its associated risks. Hypertension is a serious condition that requires close monitoring and management in order to reduce the risk of complications. With the right lifestyle changes, medical care, and monitoring, individuals can reduce their risk of developing hypertension and its associated complications.

Hypertension, also known as high blood pressure, is a serious condition that affects millions of people around the world. It occurs when the force of blood flowing through the arteries is too high, placing strain on the cardiovascular system and potentially leading to organ damage. Many of the risk factors for hypertension are lifestyle-related, such as being overweight, eating an unhealthy diet, smoking, and not getting enough physical activity. However, there are also certain medical conditions, such as kidney disease and diabetes that can increase a person's risk of developing hypertension. It is important to learn about the causes, symptoms, and treatments of hypertension, as well as how to prevent it, in order to reduce its associated risks.

Hypertension is a serious condition that requires close monitoring and management in order to reduce the risk of complications. With the right lifestyle changes, medical care, and monitoring, individuals can reduce their risk of developing hypertension and its associated complications.

With the right knowledge and care, individuals can take an active role in managing and reducing their risk of hypertension. By making small lifestyle changes, such as eating a healthy diet and exercising regularly, individuals can reduce their risk of developing hypertension and its associated complications. Additionally, it is important to talk to a doctor to discuss treatment options and to stay informed of any changes in blood pressure levels.

By understanding hypertension and taking preventative steps, individuals can live a healthier life.

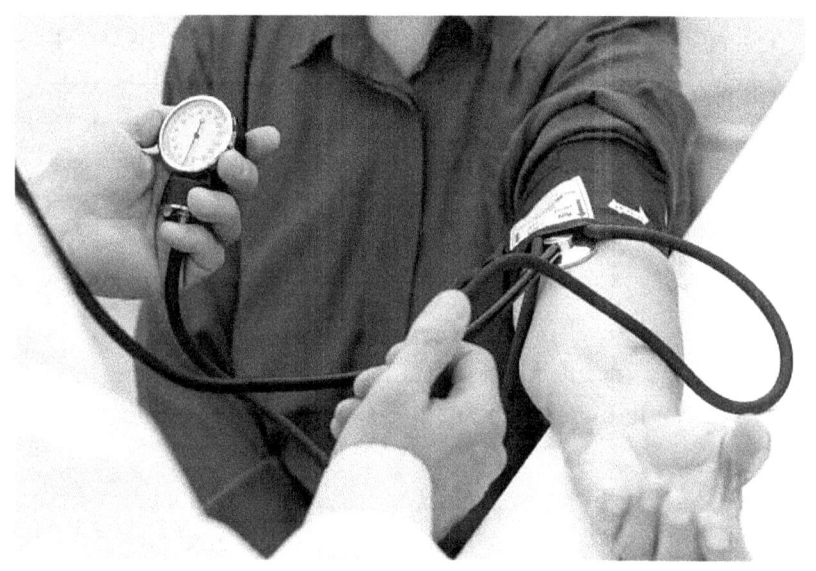

Hypertension

CHAPTER 2

Causes of Hypertension

1. Genetics: Hypertension can be hereditary, meaning it can be passed down from parents to their children. Hypertension, or high blood pressure, can be caused by a combination of genetics and environmental factors. Genetics plays a large role in the development of hypertension, as certain genes can predispose people to the condition. For example, a gene called AGT encodes a protein called angiotensinogen, which is involved in the constriction of blood vessels.

Mutations in this gene can lead to higher levels of angiotensinogen and cause the walls of the blood vessels to become more narrow and resistant to blood flow, leading to high blood pressure.

Other genes involved in hypertension include those involved in the regulation of sodium and potassium levels, as well as certain hormones, such as cortisol and aldosterone. Environmental factors, such as diet and lifestyle, can also play a role in the development of hypertension.

Genetics plays a large role in the development of hypertension, with certain genes predisposing people to the condition. Environmental factors, such as diet and lifestyle, can also contribute to the development of hypertension.

2. Diet: Eating a diet high in salt, fats, and processed foods can increase one's risk of developing hypertension.
Hypertension is a major risk factor for heart disease, stroke and other serious health conditions, and diet is a significant contributor to high blood pressure. Eating too much salt, or sodium, can cause the body to retain fluid, which increases blood pressure. Eating too much saturated and trans fat can also lead to high cholesterol, which can further contribute to hypertension. A diet high in processed, sugar-laden foods can cause weight gain, which can also raise blood pressure. Eating a healthy diet that includes plenty of fruits, vegetables, low-fat dairy, lean proteins and whole grains can help reduce your risk for hypertension.

3. Stress: Stress can contribute to a rise in blood pressure.
When a person is under stress, the body releases hormones such as adrenaline and cortisol. These hormones cause the heart to beat faster, the blood vessels to narrow, and the blood pressure to rise. Over time, this constant release of hormones can lead to high blood pressure, also known as hypertension. Hypertension can increase the risk of stroke and heart attack, and can also contribute to other health problems such as diabetes, kidney disease, and even Alzheimer's disease.
Stress can also lead to unhealthy lifestyle choices such as smoking, drinking alcohol, and overeating, all of which can

contribute to hypertension. Stress can also cause a person to become less physically active, which can lead to weight gain, a risk factor for hypertension.

4. Obstructive Sleep Apnea: This sleep disorder can cause blood pressure to spike throughout the night.

Obstructive sleep apnea is a disorder in which a person's breathing is interrupted during sleep due to a blockage of their airway. This can lead to episodes of shallow breathing or even temporary pauses in breathing, which can cause a number of physical and mental health problems, including hypertension (high blood pressure). The exact mechanism by which sleep apnea causes hypertension is not entirely understood, but it is thought to involve a combination of factors.

During an apneic episode, the body responds by sending signals to the brain to increase the heart rate and force of each heartbeat in order to bring more oxygen to the brain. This increased heart rate and force leads to increased blood pressure. Additionally, the lack of oxygen caused by the apneic episode can also lead to increased levels of stress hormones in the body, which can further increase blood pressure.

It is also thought that the body's natural circadian rhythm, or sleep-wake cycle, can be disrupted by sleep apnea, leading to decreased levels of melatonin and increased levels of cortisol. This can cause a further increase in blood pressure, as cortisol is known to increase blood pressure.

5. Smoking: Smoking can increase the risk of developing hypertension.

Smoking is a major risk factor for developing hypertension, a condition characterized by elevated blood pressure levels. People who smoke are more likely to suffer from high blood pressure than those who do not smoke. Smoking can damage the walls of the arteries, making them less flexible and less able to regulate blood pressure. This can lead to an increase in the pressure of the blood and can eventually lead to hypertension. Furthermore, smoking can cause plaque to build up in the arteries and can lead to a narrowing of the arteries, which can also increase blood pressure levels. Therefore, quitting smoking is essential for maintaining healthy blood pressure levels and reducing the risk of developing hypertension.

Also, smoking can worsen existing hypertension. Nicotine and other chemicals in cigarette smoke can increase the heart rate and cause the arteries to constrict, both of which can lead to an increase in blood pressure levels. Therefore, it is important for people who have hypertension to avoid smoking in order to prevent further damage to their cardiovascular system.

6. Obesity: Being overweight or obese can cause an increase in blood pressure.

Obesity is a major risk factor for developing hypertension, also known as high blood pressure. This is because excess weight places an additional strain on the heart, which has to work harder to pump blood around the body and maintain proper circulation. Additionally, obesity can lead to an increase in blood volume and can cause the blood vessels to become narrower, making it more difficult for blood to flow through them. This can cause elevated blood pressure, as the heart has to work harder to maintain circulation. Additionally, obesity-related changes in hormones, such as increased cortisol and insulin, can also lead to hypertension.

Obesity can also lead to other serious health conditions, such as heart disease, stroke, and diabetes. Therefore, it is important to maintain a healthy weight and lifestyle in order to reduce the risk of these conditions.

To prevent or reduce the risk of developing hypertension, it is important to maintain a healthy weight, engage in physical activity, and follow a healthy diet. Additionally, it is important to have regular check-ups with a doctor in order to monitor and manage blood pressure levels.

7. Medications: Certain medications such as birth control pills and certain decongestants can cause an increase in blood pressure.

Medication can cause hypertension in several ways. Certain medications can cause an increase in heart rate, which can lead to an increase in blood pressure. Some medications can also cause an increase in sodium retention, which can cause fluid build-up in the body, increasing blood pressure. Certain drugs, such as decongestants, can constrict the blood vessels, resulting in an increase in blood pressure. Finally, some medications can cause direct damage to the kidneys, resulting in an increase in blood pressure.

It is important to note that many medications used to treat hypertension can also cause an increase in blood pressure. Therefore, it is important to carefully monitor blood pressure when taking any medications, and to speak with a doctor or pharmacist to ensure that the medications are not causing an increase in blood pressure.

8. Age: As you age, your risk of developing hypertension increases.

Age is a major factor in the development of hypertension. As people get older, the risk of developing hypertension increases. This is due to changes in the body that occur over time. Aging can cause changes in the elasticity of the arteries, which can lead to higher blood pressure readings.

In addition, age can also affect the body's ability to regulate sodium, which can lead to an increase in blood pressure. Age-related changes in the kidneys can also contribute to hypertension. Therefore, it is important for people of all ages to monitor their blood pressure and take steps to reduce their risk of developing hypertension.

9. Gender:Men are more likely to develop hypertension than women.

Gender has been found to be a potential risk factor when it comes to the development of hypertension.

Studies have shown that men are more likely to develop hypertension than women, with men having a higher risk.

10. Alcohol consumption: Drinking large amounts of alcohol can cause an increase in blood pressure.

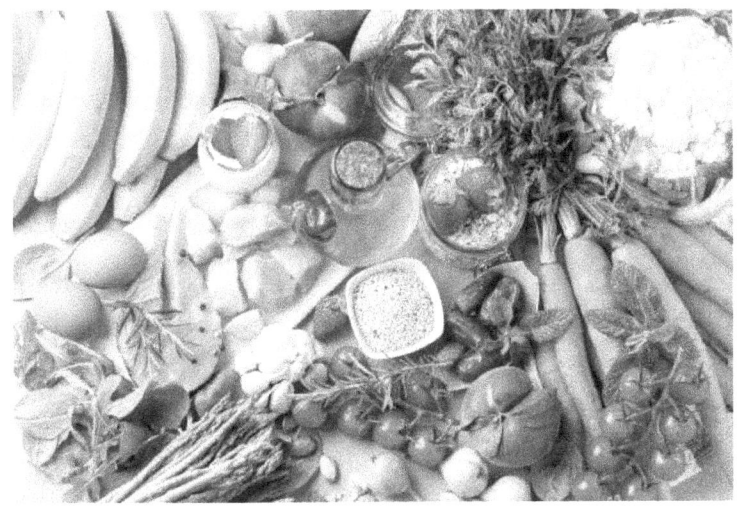

CHAPTER 3

Risk of Hypertension

1. Heart attack: Hypertension can put a strain on your heart, making it work harder than normal. This can increase your risk of a heart attack.

2. Stroke: High blood pressure can also damage the walls of your arteries, increasing the risk of a stroke.

3. Kidney damage: Long-term high blood pressure can damage the filters in your kidneys, leading to kidney failure.

4. Eye damage: High blood pressure can damage the blood vessels in your eyes, leading to vision problems.

5. Memory problems: High blood pressure can damage the blood vessels in your brain, leading to memory problems and even dementia.

6. Sexual dysfunction: Men with hypertension may experience erectile dysfunction due to damage to the blood vessels in their penis.

7. Atherosclerosis: Long-term high blood pressure can damage the walls of your arteries, leading to a build-up of plaque. This can cause atherosclerosis, which increases your risk of heart attack and stroke.

8. Pregnancy complications: High blood pressure during pregnancy can increase the risk of preterm delivery, low birth weight, and stillbirth.

9. Peripheral artery disease: High blood pressure can damage the blood vessels in your arms and legs, leading to a condition called peripheral artery disease. This can cause pain and numbness in your extremities.

10. Heart failure: Long-term high blood pressure can weaken your heart, making it less able to pump blood effectively. This can lead to heart failure.

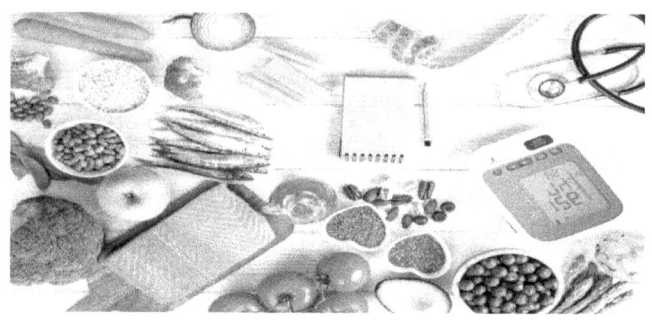

CHAPTER 4

Diagnosis and Treatment of Hypertension

Hypertension is usually diagnosed through a physical examination, including a blood pressure reading. The American College of Cardiology and the American Heart Association recommend that a diagnosis of hypertension be made if your blood pressure is consistently 140/90 mmHg or higher.

Treatment for hypertension usually involves lifestyle changes, such as exercising regularly, eating a balanced diet, and limiting alcohol and caffeine intake. In some cases, medications such as ACE inhibitors, beta-blockers, and diuretics may be prescribed. If lifestyle changes and medications do not control hypertension, a doctor may recommend further treatments such as angioplasty or surgery.

Diagnosis of hypertension includes:
1. Tests to measure your cholesterol, triglyceride and blood sugar levels
2. Tests to check for kidney disease
3. Tests to measure your pulse and heart rate
4. Tests to measure your urine sodium and creatinine levels
5. An EKG or echo to check for any structural problems in your heart
6. An ultrasound to check for any blockages in your arteries
7. A chest X-ray to check for any heart problems
8. An MRI or CT scan to check for any brain or blood vessel damage
9. Blood tests to check for any other underlying medical conditions that can cause high blood pressure

Treatment of hypertension includes:
1. Medication - Medicines such as ACE inhibitors, beta-blockers, calcium channel blockers, and diuretics can help lower your blood pressure.

2. Lifestyle changes - Eating a healthy diet, exercising regularly, limiting alcohol and caffeine intake, and reducing stress can help lower your blood pressure.

3. Weight loss - If you are overweight, losing weight can help lower your blood pressure.

4. Surgery - If lifestyle changes and medications don't work, surgery may be recommended to open blocked arteries or reduce the size of your heart.

5. Complementary therapies - Stress-reduction techniques such as meditation and yoga can help reduce your blood pressure.

It is important to follow your doctor's instructions for treating hypertension. If left untreated, hypertension can lead to serious health problems.

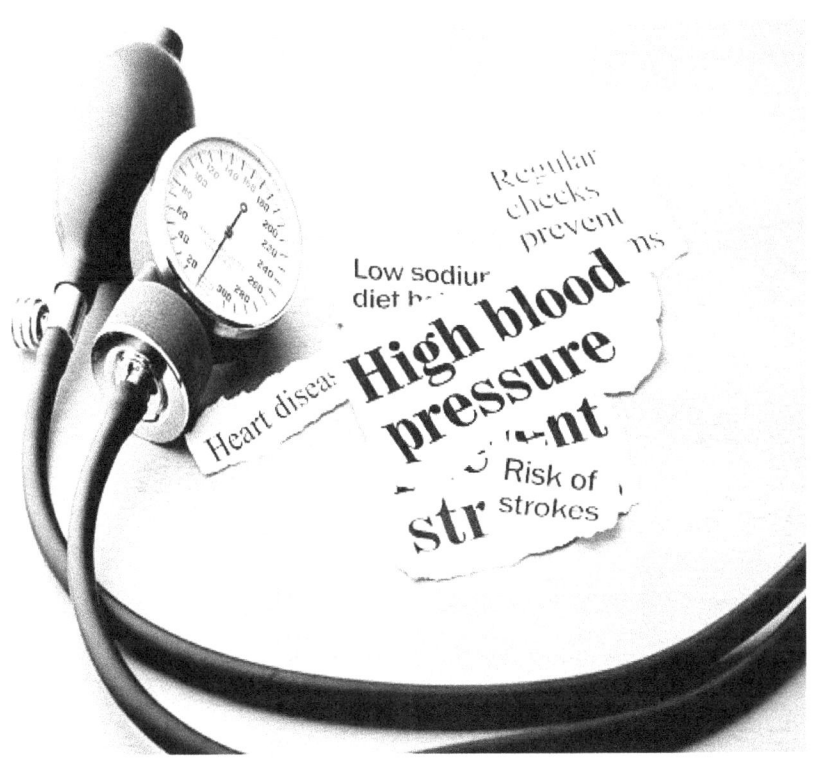

CHAPTER 5

Dietary Changes

1. Eat a diet rich in fruits, vegetables, and whole grains. Include plenty of fresh produce, such as leafy greens, cruciferous vegetables (broccoli, cauliflower), and citrus fruits.

2. Increase your intake of healthy fats, such as olive oil, nuts, avocados, and fatty fish.

3. Limit your intake of saturated fat, trans fat, and cholesterol, found in red meats, butter, and processed foods.

4. Choose lean proteins, such as poultry, fish, eggs, and legumes.

5. Reduce your intake of sodium, which is found in processed foods, canned foods, and fast foods.

6. Increase your intake of potassium, found in bananas, potatoes, and leafy greens.

7. Avoid added sugars, found in sodas, candy, and baked goods.

8. Monitor your alcohol intake and limit it to no more than one drink per day for women and two drinks per day for men.

9. Drink plenty of water to stay hydrated and to reduce your blood pressure.

10. Aim to get at least 30 minutes of physical activity on most days of the week.

CHAPTER 6

Exercise and Physical Activity

1. Swimming: Swimming is an excellent exercise for hypertensive individuals as it is low-impact and does not require joint movement. It also helps increase cardiovascular endurance and flexibility.

2. Walking: Walking is a great exercise for hypertensive individuals as it is low-impact, easy to do, and can be done anywhere. It is also an effective way to reduce stress and improve overall cardiovascular health.

3. Yoga: Yoga is a low-impact physical activity that can help relax the body and mind while strengthening the cardiovascular system. It can also reduce stress and improve overall flexibility.

4. Resistance Training: Resistance training is an effective way to build muscle mass and strengthen the cardiovascular system. It is important to always use proper form when lifting weights and start with light weights to avoid injury.

5. Cycling: Cycling is a great exercise for hypertensive individuals as it is low-impact and can be done indoors or outdoors. It helps improve cardiovascular endurance and muscular strength.

6. Tai Chi: Tai chi is a low-impact physical activity that can help reduce stress and improve flexibility. It is also an effective way to improve balance and posture.

7. Stretching: Stretching can help decrease tension in the body and improve flexibility. It can also help reduce stress and improve overall circulation.

8. Pilates: Pilates is a low-impact form of exercise that can help improve posture and reduce stress. It is also an effective way to improve strength and flexibility.

9. Aquatic Exercises: Aquatic exercises are a great way to get physical activity while reducing the risk of injury. It can also help improve cardiovascular endurance and flexibility.

10. Dancing: Dancing is a great way to get physical activity and reduce stress. It can also help improve overall body coordination and cardiovascular health.

CHAPTER 7

Stress Management and
Relaxation Techniques

These are important components of lifestyle changes and can help reduce the risk of developing hypertension. Stress hormones can increase blood pressure, so it is important to practise stress management and relaxation techniques to prevent or reduce hypertension.

Deep breathing: Deep breathing is an effective and simple relaxation technique that can be used anytime and anywhere. It helps to reduce stress, anxiety, and tension and can lower blood pressure. To practise deep breathing, find a comfortable position, close your eyes, and take a few deep breaths in through your nose and out through your mouth, focusing on the sensation of your breath.

Progressive muscle relaxation: Progressive Muscle Relaxation (PMR) is a relaxation technique that helps to reduce stress, tension, and anxiety. To practise PMR, tense and relax each muscle group in your body, starting with your head and neck and working your way down to your feet.

Meditation: Meditation is a mental and spiritual practice that helps to reduce stress, anxiety, and tension. To practise meditation, sit or lie in a comfortable position, close your eyes, and focus on your breath or a mantra.

Yoga: Yoga is a physical practice that combines stretching and breathing exercises to reduce stress, tension, and anxiety

Journaling: Journaling is a great way to express your thoughts and feelings and to reduce stress, anxiety, and tension.

Exercise: Exercise is an important component of stress management and can help to reduce stress, anxiety, and tension.

These are just a few of the stress management and relaxation techniques that can help to reduce the risk of developing hypertension. It is important to practise these techniques regularly to reduce stress and maintain a healthy lifestyle.

CHAPTER 8

Monitoring and Managing Hypertension

Monitoring and managing hypertension is important for the prevention of many long-term health complications. It is important to monitor blood pressure levels regularly and to make lifestyle changes to help manage the condition.

In terms of monitoring, it is important to measure blood pressure levels at least every two years. If levels are consistently high, it is important to see a doctor for further testing and to confirm the diagnosis. It is also important to keep track of any changes in levels and to report any sudden spikes or dips in blood pressure to a doctor.

In terms of managing hypertension, lifestyle changes are essential. This includes eating a healthy diet, exercising regularly, reducing stress, and limiting alcohol consumption. Additionally, it is important to take medications as prescribed and to monitor their effectiveness. It is also important to be aware of any potential side effects of the medications and to contact a doctor if any occur.

By monitoring and managing hypertension, it is possible to reduce the risk of long-term health complications and to improve overall health and quality of life.

Monitoring and managing hypertension is important for the prevention of many long-term health complications. It is important to monitor blood pressure levels regularly and to make lifestyle changes to help manage the condition.
In terms of monitoring, it is important to measure blood pressure levels at least every two years. If levels are consistently high, it is important to see a doctor for further testing and to confirm the diagnosis. It is also important to keep track of any changes in levels and to report any sudden spikes or dips in blood pressure to a doctor.

In terms of managing hypertension, lifestyle changes are essential. This includes eating a healthy diet, exercising regularly, reducing stress, and limiting alcohol consumption. Additionally, it is important to take medications as prescribed and to monitor their effectiveness. It is also important to be aware of any potential side effects of the medications and to contact a doctor if any occur.
By monitoring and managing hypertension, it is possible to reduce the risk of long-term health complications and to improve overall health and quality of life.

Ensure you

• Monitor your blood pressure levels at least every two years

• Make lifestyle changes, such as eating a healthy diet, exercising regularly, reducing stress, and limiting alcohol consumption

• Take prescribed medications and monitor their effectiveness

• Be aware of the potential side effects of medications and contact a doctor if any occur

On Monitoring and Managing Hypertension

• Follow up with your doctor regularly to ensure that your treatment plan is working properly

• Stay informed about the latest research and recommendations on hypertension management

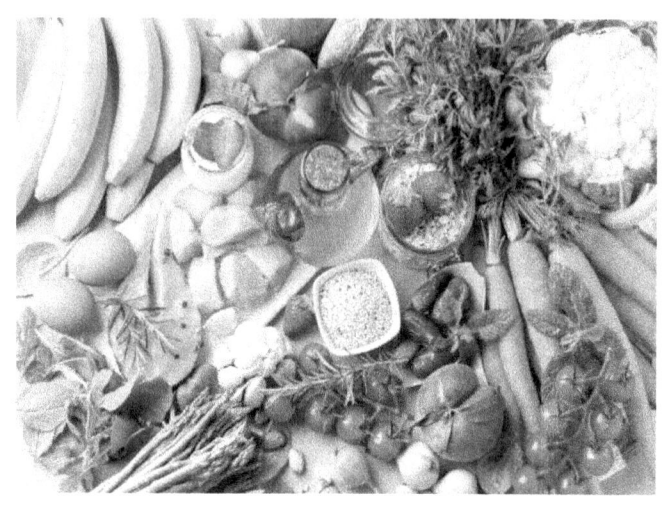

CHAPTER 9

Hypertensive meal plan

The following is a recommended meal plan and recipes for patients with high blood pressure.

DAY 1

Breakfast:

Oatmeal Pancakes

Ingredients:

-1/2 cup rolled oats
-1/4 cup all-purpose flour
-1/4 teaspoon baking soda
-1/4 teaspoon baking powder
-1/4 teaspoon salt
-1/2 cup low-fat milk
-1 egg
-1 tablespoon honey
-1 teaspoon butter
-1/4 teaspoon ground cinnamon

Procedure:

1. In a medium bowl, mix together the oats, flour, baking soda, baking powder, and salt.

2. In a separate bowl, whisk together the milk, egg, honey, butter, and cinnamon until combined.

3. Add the wet ingredients to the dry ingredients and stir until just combined.

4. Heat a non-stick skillet over medium heat.

5. Grease the skillet with a small amount of butter.

6. Drop the batter onto the skillet in 1/4 cup portions.

7. Cook until the edges are brown and bubbles form on the top.

8. Flip the pancakes and cook until both sides are golden brown.

9. Serve with fresh fruit or maple syrup.

Lunch:

Avocado Toast

Ingredients:

-2 slices of whole-wheat bread
-1 ripe avocado
-1/4 teaspoon garlic powder
-1/4 teaspoon ground cumin
-1/4 teaspoon paprika
-Salt and pepper, to taste
-1/4 cup crumbled feta cheese
-1 tablespoon fresh parsley, chopped

Procedure:

1. Toast the bread slices until golden brown.

2. Mash the avocado in a bowl.

3. Add the garlic powder, cumin, paprika, salt, and pepper.

4. Spread the avocado mixture onto the toast.

5. Top with feta cheese and parsley.

6. Serve immediately.

Dinner:

Roasted Salmon with Asparagus

Ingredients:

-1/2 pound salmon
-1/2 lemon, sliced
-2 tablespoons olive oil
-1/2 teaspoon garlic powder

-1/2 teaspoon paprika
-Salt and pepper, to taste
-1 pound asparagus, trimmed

Procedure:

1. Preheat the oven to 400°F.

2. Line a baking sheet with parchment paper.

3. Place the salmon on the parchment paper.

4. Top with lemon slices.

5. Drizzle with olive oil and sprinkle with garlic powder, paprika, salt, and pepper.

6. Place the asparagus on the baking sheet and drizzle with olive oil.

7. Bake for 15-20 minutes, or until the salmon is cooked through and the asparagus is tender.

Write a week meal plan for hypertensive patient with the cooking procedure

DAY 2

Breakfast:
Overnight oats with blueberries
Cooking procedure: In a bowl, combine 1/2 cup of rolled oats, 1/2 cup of milk, 1/4 cup of Greek yogurt, 1 tablespoon

of chia seeds, and a handful of blueberries. Cover and refrigerate overnight. Serve the next morning.

Lunch: Avocado and tomato salad
Cooking procedure: Slice 1 avocado and 1 tomato and place in a bowl. Add in 1/4 cup of diced red onion, 2 tablespoons of olive oil, 1 tablespoon of lemon juice, and salt and pepper to taste. Mix together until combined.

Snack: Apple slices with almond butter
Cooking procedure: Slice an apple into thin slices and spread a tablespoon of almond butter on each slice.

Dinner: Baked tilapia with roasted potatoes
Cooking procedure: Preheat oven to 375F.

Toss cubed potatoes with a tablespoon of olive oil, salt, and pepper. Place potatoes on a baking sheet and bake for 25 minutes. Meanwhile, season tilapia fillets with salt and pepper and place on a baking sheet. Bake for 15 minutes. Serve the tilapia with roasted potatoes.

DAY 3

Breakfast: Greek yogurt parfait with granola
Cooking procedure: Layer Greek yogurt, granola, and fresh berries in a bowl.

Lunch: Grilled chicken wrap with vegetables
Cooking procedure: Heat a grill or grill pan to medium-high heat and add a tablespoon of oil. Grill chicken until cooked through, about 4-5 minutes per side. Remove from heat and slice into strips. Place the chicken strips in a wrap with lettuce, tomatoes, and cucumbers.

Snack: Celery and peanut butter
Cooking procedure: Spread a tablespoon of peanut butter on celery sticks.

Dinner: Broiled cod with roasted asparagus
Cooking procedure: Preheat oven to broil. Place cod fillets on a baking sheet and season with salt and pepper. Broil for 8-10 minutes. Meanwhile, toss asparagus with a tablespoon of olive oil, salt, and pepper. Place on a baking sheet and broil for 8 minutes. Serve the cod with the roasted asparagus.

DAY 4

Breakfast: Smoothie bowl with banana and berries
Cooking procedure: Blend 1 banana, 1/2 cup of frozen berries, 1/2 cup
Of yogurt, and 1/4 cup of milk until smooth. Pour into a bowl and top with sliced banana and fresh berries.

Lunch: Turkey and spinach wrap
Cooking procedure: Spread a tablespoon of hummus on a wrap and top with turkey slices, spinach, and tomatoes.

Snack: Cucumber slices with cottage cheese
Cooking procedure: Slice a cucumber into thin slices and top with 1/4 cup of cottage cheese.

Dinner: Baked chicken with quinoa and roasted vegetables
Cooking procedure: Preheat oven to 425F. Season a chicken breast with salt and pepper and place in an oven-safe dish. Roast for 20 minutes. Meanwhile, cook quinoa according to package instructions. Toss sliced carrots, onions, and bell peppers with a tablespoon of olive oil, salt, and pepper. Place vegetables on a baking sheet and roast for 25 minutes. Serve the roasted chicken with quinoa and roasted vegetables.

DAY 5

Breakfast: Oatmeal with banana
Cooking procedure: Place 1/2 cup of rolled oats, 1 cup of water, and a pinch of salt in a pot. Bring to a boil, reduce heat to low, and simmer for 5 minutes.

Lunch: Grilled vegetable wrap

Cooking procedure: Heat a grill or grill pan to medium-high heat and add a tablespoon of oil. Grill sliced bell peppers, zucchini, eggplant, and onions until tender, about 4-5 minutes per side. Place the vegetables in a wrap with lettuce, tomato, and cucumbers.

Snack: Greek yogurt with almonds
Cooking procedure: Top 1/2 cup of Greek yogurt with a handful of almonds.

Dinner: Baked salmon with roasted broccoli
Cooking procedure: Preheat oven to 425F. Season salmon fillets with salt and pepper and place on a baking sheet. Roast for 15 minutes. Meanwhile, toss broccoli florets with a tablespoon of olive oil, salt, and pepper. Place on a baking sheet and roast for 15 minutes. Serve the baked salmon with the roasted broccoli.

DAY 6

Breakfast: Toast with peanut butter and banana
Cooking procedure: Toast 2 slices of bread. Spread each slice with a tablespoon of peanut butter and top with 1/2 banana, sliced.

Lunch: Quinoa bowl with roasted vegetables

Cooking procedure: Cook quinoa according to package instructions. Preheat oven to 425F. Toss sliced carrots, onions, and bell peppers with a tablespoon of olive oil, salt, and pepper. Place vegetables on a baking sheet and roast for 25 minutes. Serve the quinoa with the roasted vegetables.

Snack: Celery and hummus
Cooking procedure: Spread 2 tablespoons of hummus on celery sticks.

Dinner: Grilled shrimp with roasted sweet potato
Cooking procedure: Preheat oven to 425F. Peel and dice a sweet potato and toss with a tablespoon of olive oil, salt, and pepper. Place on a baking sheet and roast for 25 minutes. Meanwhile, heat a grill or grill pan to medium-high heat and add a tablespoon of oil. Grill shrimp until cooked through, about 2-3 minutes per side. Serve the grilled shrimp with the roasted sweet potato.

DAY 7

Breakfast: Avocado toast with a fried
Cooking procedure: Toast 2 slices of bread. Spread each slice with 1/2 avocado and top with a fried egg.

Lunch: Baked salmon with roasted broccoli

Cooking procedure: Preheat oven to 425F. Season salmon fillets with salt and pepper and place on a baking sheet. Roast for 15 minutes. Meanwhile, toss broccoli florets with a tablespoon of olive oil, salt, and pepper. Place on a baking sheet and roast for 15 minutes. Serve the baked salmon with the roasted broccoli.

Snack: Apple slices with almond butter
Cooking procedure: Slice an apple into thin slices and spread a tablespoon of almond butter on each slice.

Dinner: Grilled chicken with roasted potatoes
Cooking procedure: Heat a grill or grill pan to medium-high heat and add a tablespoon of oil. Grill chicken until cooked through, about 4-5 per side. Meanwhile, toss cubed potatoes with a tablespoon of olive oil, salt, and pepper. Place potatoes on a baking sheet and bake for 25 minutes. Serve the grilled chicken with the roasted potatoes.